HIDDEN REMEDIES

Cancer & Other Illnesses

By Rene Jackson

ISBN: 9798863760261

Table of Contents

Introduction 2

Chapter One: Cancer.. 3

Ozone Therapy for Cancer 4

Leech Therapy for Cancer 6

Vitamin C Therapy for Cancer 8

Acupuncture for Cancer 10

Cupping for Cancer 12

Ruqya for Cancer 15

Other Methods for Treating Cancer 17

Chapter Two: Herpes.. 19

A Doctor from Honduras 20

A Breakthrough from Australia............................ 26

A New Product in America 31

Glad Tidings from the Mideast 34

An Approach Rarely Thought Of 39

Methods to Control the Virus 45

About the Author.. 49

Introduction

Diseases that were unheard of a thousand years ago are now becoming widespread. Cancer, HIV, and herpes, to name a few. Unfortunately, for many of these ailments, a cure has yet to be discovered. Or has it? Perhaps not officially, but there are those who claim to have discovered a cure for uncurable diseases such as cancer and herpes.

Though it's against FDA guidelines to claim a cure for such diseases, there are companies around the world- outside of FDA's jurisdictions- that have carried out their own research and have formulated successful treatments for cancer, diabetes, and herpes.

In this book, we will take a glance at proven methods which have been used to completely cure cancer, diabetes, and even herpes. Some testimonials will be shared as well as resources so that you or your loved one may avail of services provided around the world. We do recommend that you do detailed research before deciding which treatment you may wish to undertake.

I myself have personally suffered from some ailments which were deemed incurable, but God decreed otherwise for me. I will share this with you later in the book.

CHAPTER ONE

CANCER

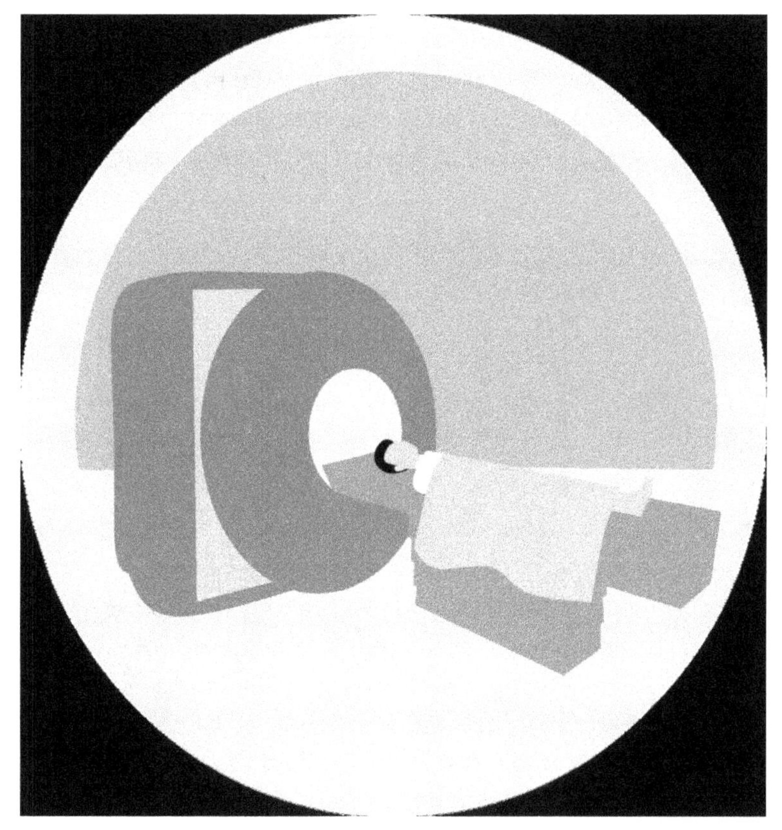

Ozone Therapy for Cancer

What is Ozone Therapy?

People suffering from cancer are oftentimes presented with three options as a remedy for their cancer- surgery, chemotherapy, or radiation, among others. Though I was diagnosed with cancer and was presented with radiation as an option, I chose not to pursue it. Why not? From what it seems to me (**in my opinion**), is that people who undergo chemotherapy and radiation seem to be hastened to their death.

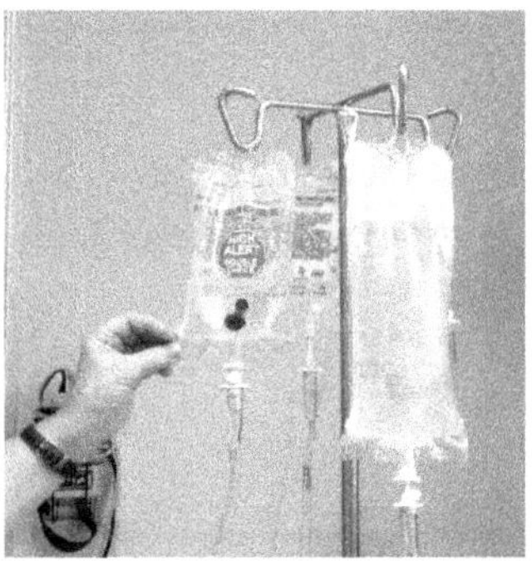

One alternative method used to treat cancer, (and sometimes used in conjunction with chemotherapy and radiation) is Ozone Therapy. Ozone Therapy has become popular in recent years, especially in Europe, where the procedure can be done at a nominal price. It entails extracting the blood by way of an IV and mixing it with Ozone and then recirculating it back to the bloodstream. The procedure lasts approximately 30 minutes. It is believed that Ozone Therapy can result in the death of cancerous cells.

Where can I get Ozone Therapy?

Though you may find some centers in America that offer Ozone Therapy, it is not as widespread as it is in Turkey. A Google search in English or in Turkish (using Google translate) will show many places that offer this therapy. Prices are extremely cheap in comparison to western countries. You will also find some providers in the UK.

Leech Therapy for Cancer

What is Leech Therapy?

Leech therapy is as the name implies. It entails using leeches to treat a patient. Since ancient times, leeches have been used to treat a number of ailments, from skin diseases, infections, arthritis, diabetes, cardiovascular disease, and even cancer. One to several leeches are placed on a patient, in the affected area and left there for several minutes (20 -45), allowing the leeches to suck the patient's blood. No worries, it doesn't hurt.

Leech therapy is sometimes used for symptomatic relief of pain in cancer patients. One academic journal reported that a 62-year-old with pain related to cancer was pain free after 2 months of leech therapy.[1] Please note that it may not be advisable for **blood** cancer patients to undergo Leech Therapy.

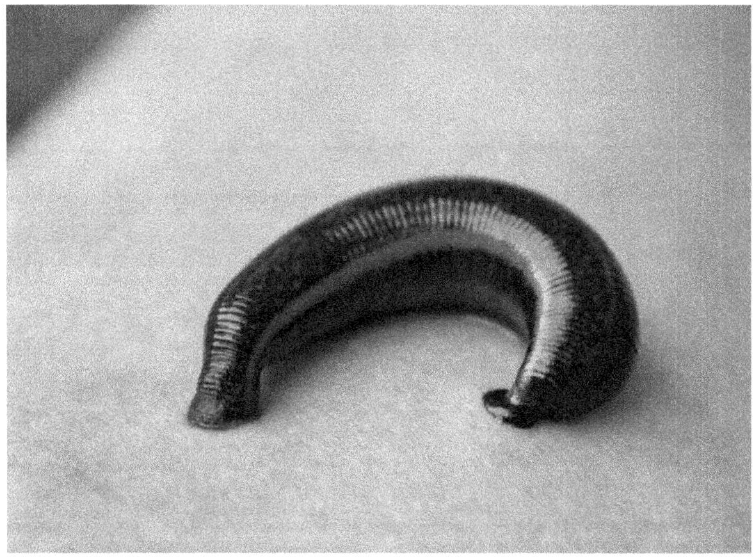

Where can I get Leech Therapy?

---

[1] (Pain Medicine, Volume 11, Issue 3, March 2010, Pages 443-445).

As with Ozone Therapy, you can find many medical centers in Turkey that offer this service at a very reasonable price. There are also a few centers in the United States, UK, and India.

I've had this done, and it doesn't hurt. It just gives you a creepy feeling seeing a bunch of live insects on your body. You do feel great afterwards though! A real cleanse.

Vitamin C Therapy for Cancer

What is Vitamin C Therapy?

We all are familiar with Vitamin C and know that we can get it from citrus fruit such as oranges and lemons. What may be new to you, however, is that Vitamin C is sometimes given in large doses for a variety of reasons. In addition to boosting the immune system and warding off a cold, Vitamin C infused intravenously is also good for neurological diseases, depression, fatigue, and even cancer.

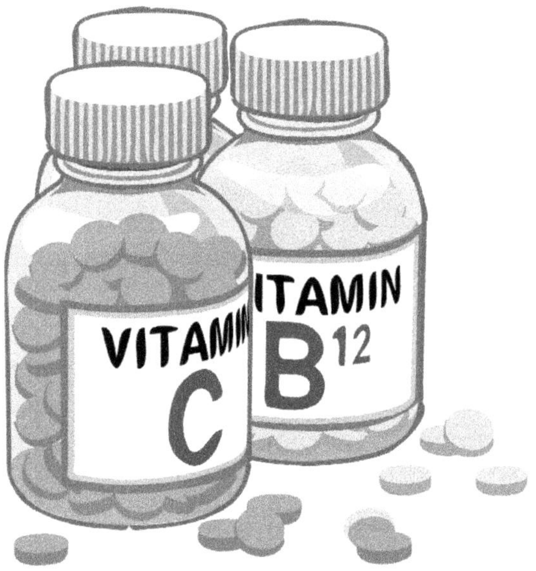

On the National Cancer Institute website, the official website of the United States government, several studies were disclosed in which Vitamin C therapy was given to pancreatic cancer and colorectal cancer patients. This was done in conjunction with chemotherapy or following it. Results were favorable for those who underwent the Vitamin C Therapy. [2]

Where can I get Vitamin C Therapy?

Unlike the other therapies previously mentioned, Vitamin C Therapy is pretty common. It can be found in Alternative Medicine practices in the United States and United Kingdom. Turkey, of course, offers it in many locations throughout the country. It is offered in India as well.

----

[2] National Cancer Institute, cancer.gov, Intravenous Vitamin C, Patient Version

Acupuncture for Cancer

What is Acupuncture?

Acupuncture is a traditional Chinese medical approach which entails inserting thin needles in affected parts of the body. When the needle is inserted, you barely feel it. It looks scarier than it actually is. When I had it done, prior to the onset of pain from my cancer, it did not hurt. However, later, when the needles were placed in the location of my pain, it caused me more pain, so I stopped my treatment.

Acupuncture has many benefits. It's known to treat arthritis, Carpal Tunnel Syndrome, fatigue, and PD (Parkinson's Disease). According to the Science Direct Journal, "acupuncture has a high potential to become a prominent treatment option for PD." [3]

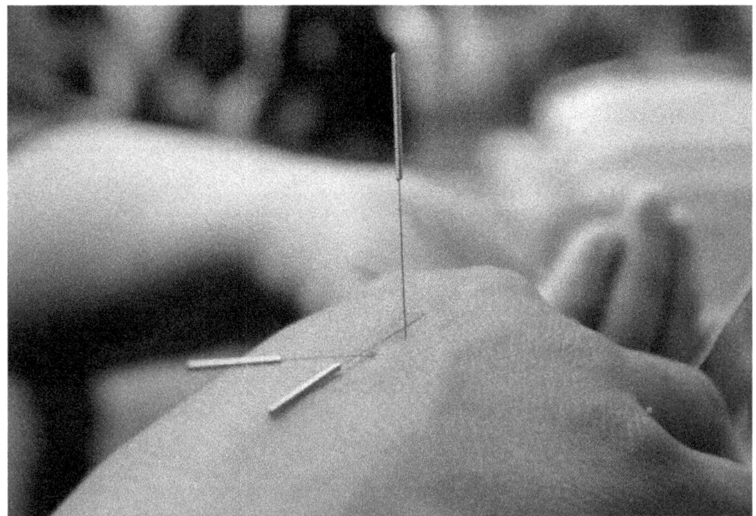

---

[3] Science Direct Journal, "Acupuncture for Parkinson's Disease: From Theory to Practice. https://www.sciencedirect.com/

Though it didn't suit me well, acupuncture is actually used to relieve pain- back pain, neck pain, headaches, menstrual cramps, and even pain from cancer. According to the National Library of Medicine, some cancer centers in America are using acupuncture to treat cancer and find it especially effective for those undergoing chemotherapy. It is said to assist with removing nausea, vomiting, pain, and fatigue associated with cancer.[4]

Where can I get Acupuncture?

Though originally practiced by the Chinese, acupuncture can now be found almost anywhere.

---

[4] National Library of Medicine, "The Value of Acupuncture in Cancer Care" https://www.ncbi.nlm.nih.gov/pmc/articles/PMC2642987/

Cupping for Cancer

What is Cupping?

Cupping is a method of treatment in which suction cups are applied to a particular part of the body- usually the back, to help release toxins from that area. It is a practice that has been implemented by the Chinese for thousands of years. It is also a tradition that is done in the Muslim world and was highly recommended by Prophet Muhammad (Peace be upon him and on all the other prophets) more than 1400 years ago.

The Chinese usually use heat (fire) before applying the cups. Muslims, on the other hand, often do wet cupping (known as hijama), which entails applying the suction cups for several minutes then using a razon to make small cuts. The cups are then applied again for another several minutes, causing the bad blood to flow out of the area where the cuts were made. Do the slits hurt? No, they don't if it's done correctly.

Alternatively, sometimes practitioners do cupping massage, which is dry cupping combined with massaging the area with the cups and sometimes with the hands.

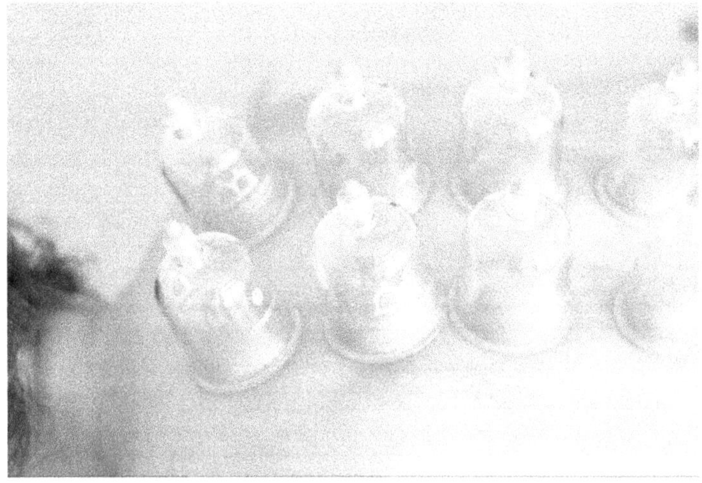

What are the benefits of cupping? Cupping has many benefits. In addition to releasing toxins from the body, cupping is good for patients suffering from the following ailments:

- high blood pressure

- arthritis

- anxiety

- depression

- diabetes

- herpes

- cancer

Cupping is helpful to diabetes patients because it releases the toxins in the blood, thus improving blood circulation. Both dry cupping and wet cupping have proven beneficial.[5]

Wet cupping for herpes is a therapy traditionally used by the Chinese. According to the National Library of Medicine, studies show that wet cupping was found to be effective in treating herpes.[6]

As for cancer, results from a study showed that symptoms from cancer were relieved after cupping.[7] My son, who does cupping, had a cancer patient who relayed to him that his doctor was surprised at his progress after having received cupping every 3 weeks.

---

[5] National Library of Medicine, "Hijama (Wet Cupping or Dry Cupping) for Diabetes Treatment" https://www.ncbi.nlm.nih.gov
[6] National Library of Medicine, "Wet Cupping for Therapy for Treatment of Herpes Zoster" https://www.ncbi.nlm.nih.gov
[7] National Library of Medicine, "Cupping Therapy as an Adjunctive Therapy for Side Effects of Colorectal Cancer Treatment" https://www.ncbi.nlm.nih.gov

Where can I get Cupping done?

Like acupuncture, cupping is found practically everywhere. A Google search is all that is needed to find a practitioner. To find cupping in the Muslim community, simply type the words 'hijama near me' in the search.

Ruqya for Cancer

What is Ruqya?

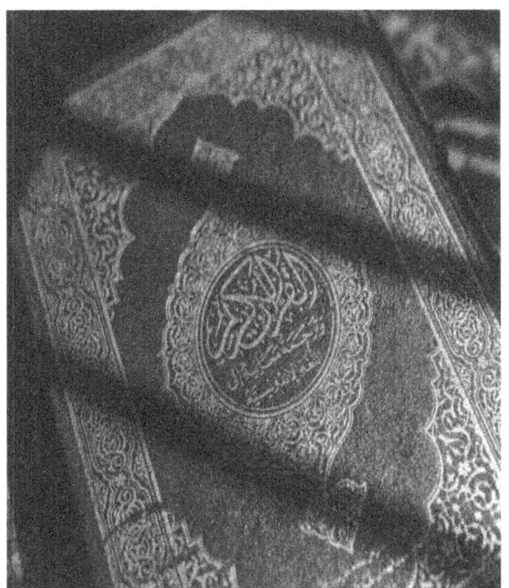

Ruqya is a method of treatment in which the Holy Quran is recited over a patient. The Quran is the last Divine revelation that was revealed to Prophet Muhammad (Peace be upon him), the last prophet, over 1400 years ago. It is a Book that contains laws by which billions of Muslims around the world follow. It's recited daily in the prayers and outside of prayers by those seeking nearness to the Creator.

One way in which the Quran is used outside of the prayer is to treat a person afflicted with an illness such as insect bites, jinn possession, cancer, and other illnesses.

"Some of the companions of the Prophet Muhammad (Peace be upon him) came across a tribe amongst the tribes of the Arabs, and that tribe did not entertain them. While they were in that state, the chief of that tribe was bitten by a snake (or stung by a scorpion). They said, (to the companions of the Prophet (ﷺ)), 'Have you got any medicine with you or anybody who can treat with Ruqya?' The Prophet's companions said, 'You refuse to entertain us, so we will not treat (your chief) unless you pay us for it.' So they agreed to pay them a flock of sheep. One of them (the Prophet's companions) started reciting Surat-al-Fatiha and gathering his saliva and spitting it (at the snake-bite). The patient got cured and his people presented the sheep to them, but they said, 'We will not take it unless we ask the Prophet (whether it is lawful).' When they asked him, he smiled and said, 'How do you know that Surat-al-Fatiha is a Ruqya? Take it (flock of sheep) and assign a share for me."[8]

Many Muslim experts who specialize in treating jinn possession cases say that many cancer cases are due to jinn (evil spirit) possession. Thus, you will find some cancer patients seeking ruqya treatment.

Where can I get ruqya done?

Most Islamic centers can refer you to someone who knows how to recite Quran over a sick patient.

---

[8] Sahih Bukhari, Volume 7, Book 71, Number 632

Other Methods for Treating Cancer

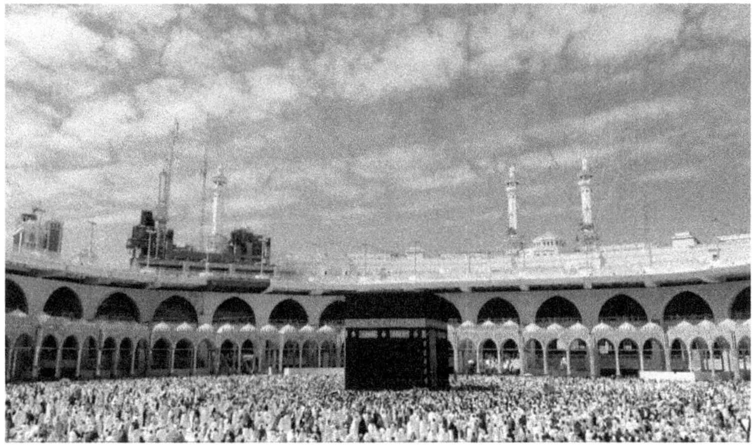

What other alternative methods are there for treating cancer?

Some other methods that you may never have heard of are:

- **Umrah/Hajj**- Hajj is the annual pilgrimage to Saudi Arabia that Muslims should make once in a life time, if able. It consists of various rituals, all of which focus on getting closer to the Creator and seeking His forgiveness. Umrah is a lesser pilgrimage, which can be done at any time. People have gone on both pilgrimages with major ailments and returned cured. Type 'Allah Removes the Cancer' on YouTube to listen to a moving success story.

- **Zam Zam Water**- Many Muslims also seek a cure by drinking Zam Zam water, which is from a well that miraculously sprang up for Hajar, Prophet Abraham's wife, when she had nothing to drink.

- **Camel Urine**- This may sound surprising, but drinking camel urine mixed with camel milk was recommended by the last Prophet, Muhammad over 1400 years ago as a cure (Peace be upon him). It has been used in recent times as a proven cure for cancer. Enter the following words in YouTube to find a sheikh sharing a success story of a friend of his (cured cancer camel urine sheikh assim).

- **Graviola-** Also known as soursop, Graviola is a fruit tree that has many benefits. Not only does it have antiviral properties, thus making it effective against herpes, but it also is known to reduce blood pressure and fight cancer. Studies have been done in which Graviola was shown to reduce or eliminate tumors.[9]

- **Boswellia-** If you're familiar with Frankincense incense, then you know Boswellia. It's an herbal extract taken from the same tree in which Frankincense incense is made. Among the benefits of Boswellia are that it is useful in curing arthritis, Parkinson's disease, asthma, and even cancer. Studies have shown that Boswellia may stop cancer growth.[10]

- **Turmeric-** We all are familiar with the spice that turns our rice yellow. Not only is turmeric used in the kitchen, but it is also used for curing ailments such as heart disease, Alzheimer's, arthritis, and even cancer. Studies have shown that turmeric can prevent cancer and kill cancer cells as well.[11]

---

[9] Graviola for Cancer Treatment: Benefits and Risks.
https://www.webmd.com/cancer/graviola-cancer-overview

[10] https://www.healthline.com/health/boswellia#cancer
https://www.medicalnewstoday.com/articles/326599#how-to-take

[11] "10 Proven Health Benefits of Turmeric and Curcumin"
www.healthline.com/nutrition

CHAPTER TWO

HERPES

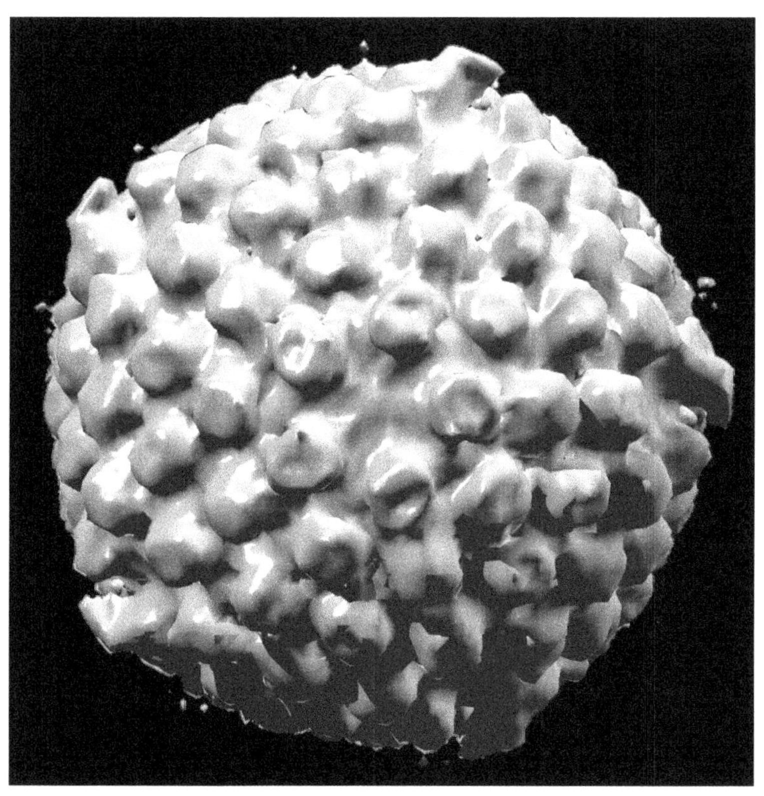

A Doctor from Honduras: Dr. Sebi

Who is Dr. Sebi?

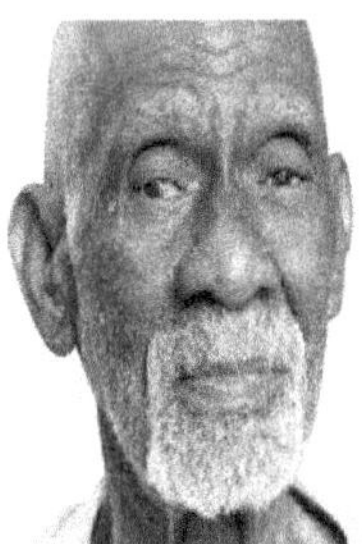

Dr. Sebi, born with the name Alfredo Bowman, was a world-renowned herbalist. He was born on November 26, 1933, in a village in Honduras. At a young age, he learned a lot about natural cures from his grandmother "Mama Hay". Though he never had a formal education, he earned the title 'Doctor' because of his extensive knowledge of herbs.

His journey on the path of seeking knowledge in natural cures began with his grandmother and continued after he met an herbalist in Mexico. Dr. Sebi had diabetes and was grossly overweight, but after the guidance of the Mexican herbalist, he lost weight and regained good health. Some years later, Dr. Sebi and his wife began treating people afflicted with various ailments free of charge. Dr. Sebi became known as a healer who treated diseases that were deemed uncurable. He would often take trips to his hometown to get herbs which he used to make his herbal formulas.

In May of 2016, Dr. Sebi made his last trip to his native country, Honduras. While there, Dr. Sebi was arrested for money laundering. Three months later, while still in custody, Dr. Sebi, loved by people all around the world, died at the age of 82. Dr. Sebi is still known and respected for having promoted a plant-based alkaline diet. Many of his videos can be found on YouTube.

Testimonials

Dr. Sebi was arrested in 1987 and charged with practicing without a license. He was also accused of making false claims of being able to cure the uncurable. Though told to present nine witnesses to support his claims, Dr. Sebi presented 77 cases present in court, all with documentation to show that they were indeed free of their major health issues after following Dr. Sebi's herbal and dietary recommendations. Dr. Sebi was therefore acquitted of the charge.

Among the celebrities who sought Dr. Sebi's treatment, were Michael Jackson, Lisa 'Left Eye' Lopez, Eddie Murphy, and John Travolta.

His Products

Dr. Sebi established a practice in California where he sold products to people around the world. That practice is now run by non-family members. Unfortunately, there is some conflict between that business and some family members, who have set up their own businesses as well. Some claim that the products sold there are no longer the original. If you would like to order from that store, you can visit the link below. The first link leads to the main page and the second one to where special packages are ordered for those who have herpes and other major illnesses. You can call the office to seek their advice first before deciding which package to choose.

https://drsebiscellfood.com/

https://drsebiscellfood.com/collections/packages

Dr. Sebi's Office, Inc

2807 La Cienega Avenue Los Angeles, CA 90034

310-838-2490

info@drsebiscellfood.com
Monday-Friday

9:00 AM - 12:30 PM

1:30 PM - 5:00 PM

All times are pacific time.

In addition to the California practice, Dr. Sebi also used to treat patients at Usha Village in Honduras. Patients stay for at least one week to treat their ailments, and they have access to geothermal waters, a natural sauna, herbal packages, and daily meals that help eradicate their diseases.

https://ushavillagehn.com/

Recommended Diet

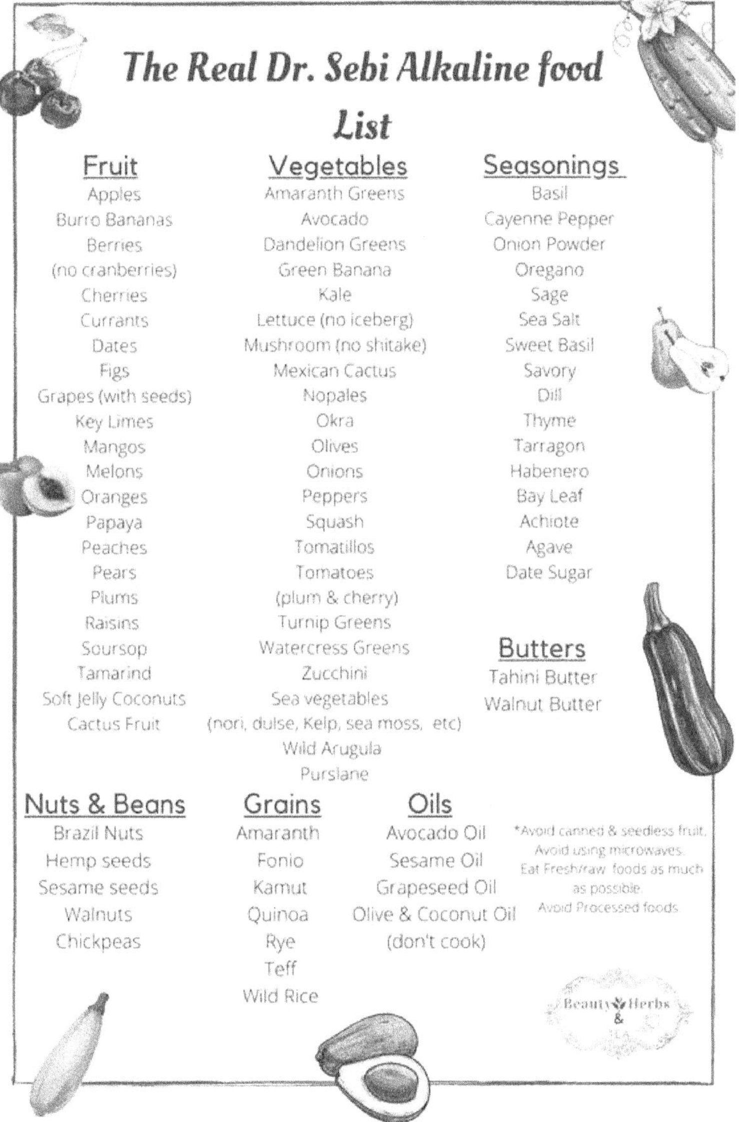

The Real Dr. Sebi Alkaline food List

Fruit
Apples
Burro Bananas
Berries
(no cranberries)
Cherries
Currants
Dates
Figs
Grapes (with seeds)
Key Limes
Mangos
Melons
Oranges
Papaya
Peaches
Pears
Plums
Raisins
Soursop
Tamarind
Soft Jelly Coconuts
Cactus Fruit

Vegetables
Amaranth Greens
Avocado
Dandelion Greens
Green Banana
Kale
Lettuce (no iceberg)
Mushroom (no shitake)
Mexican Cactus
Nopales
Okra
Olives
Onions
Peppers
Squash
Tomatillos
Tomatoes
(plum & cherry)
Turnip Greens
Watercress Greens
Zucchini
Sea vegetables
(nori, dulse, Kelp, sea moss, etc)
Wild Arugula
Purslane

Seasonings
Basil
Cayenne Pepper
Onion Powder
Oregano
Sage
Sea Salt
Sweet Basil
Savory
Dill
Thyme
Tarragon
Habenero
Bay Leaf
Achiote
Agave
Date Sugar

Butters
Tahini Butter
Walnut Butter

Nuts & Beans
Brazil Nuts
Hemp seeds
Sesame seeds
Walnuts
Chickpeas

Grains
Amaranth
Fonio
Kamut
Quinoa
Rye
Teff
Wild Rice

Oils
Avocado Oil
Sesame Oil
Grapeseed Oil
Olive & Coconut Oil
(don't cook)

*Avoid canned & seedless fruit.
Avoid using microwaves.
Eat Fresh/raw foods as much
as possible.
Avoid Processed foods.

Beauty Herbs & Tea

Dr. Sebi's Wives

It has been said that Dr. Sebi had several wives and 17 children.

Maa Bowman, his wife of 30 years, worked alongside him in developing the initial products. She set up a business many years ago while Dr. Sebi was alive and called it Fig tree Bio Electric. The link to her website is below.

https://figtreebio.com/

Before placing your order, I do advise you to reach out to them first to confirm they are taking orders, as there have been complaints of people not receiving their orders.

Patsy Bowman is the last reported legal wife of Dr. Sebi. She worked alongside him for over 20 years, assisting him with developing herbal formulas. In recent years, she started a website called *International Healing* in which she also sells Dr. Sebi's products. On her website, she makes a recommendation for sufferers of the herpes virus. She suggests that they purchase the *Intercellular Therapy Package* and states, that "this package will last for one month of treatment. After 1 month, you are either completely cured of the ailment or your viral load has decreased. If you are cured, you are done with the program; if not, then the viral load has decreased, and you need to order another package until it is eradicated. Either way, you will see results, and we ask that you get tested after the month to see where you stand."

The link to her website is listed below.

https://www.intlherbalproducts.com/

Pros & Cons

One advantage of ordering from Dr. Sebi's line of products is that, in the past, it was proven to work in completely eradicating the virus from the system. The cons, on the other hand, are that there are ongoing disputes between the three companies, each claiming to have the original formula and alleging that the others do not. In addition, the products can be quite expensive. Packages are several hundred dollars.

To reduce the burden on customers, the California office now has *Klarna* on their website, which allows qualifying customers to pay in four interest-free installments.

A Breakthrough from Australia: Synergy Pharmaceuticals

Who are they?

Hailing out of Australia is a pharmaceutical company which started in 2007. Synergy Pharmaceuticals is a reputable company in Australia which, in the past, was invited to present at international medical conferences in Japan and Canada. They have always had as its goal to help patients achieve optimal health. After spending many years researching the effects the herpes virus has on the body, Synergy Pharmaceuticals developed a comprehensive treatment to eliminate the virus from the body. Their success rate is 70 percent.

Products

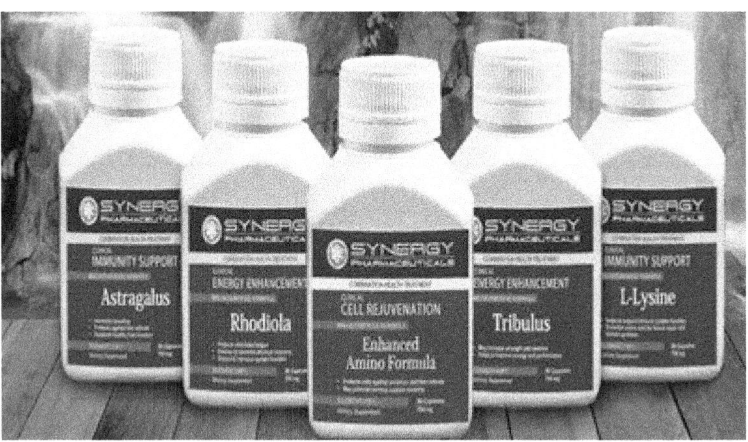

Synergy provides five different herbs for customers suffering from the herpes virus. Their products are all plant-based and are non-GMO. Not only are they good for herpes sufferers, but they are great for boosting the immune system. One satisfied customer stated, "You can cough in my face, and I still won't get sick (while taking these herbs)."

Synergy recommends that customers take the herbs for 4 to 6 months to eliminate the herpes virus from the system. They have posted before and after test results of some of their customers on their website. Products are available as a one-month supply, three months, or six months' supply. Prices range from $79 to $318 but are often on sale for as low as $49 for a one-month supply.

The ingredients contained in their products are listed below.

Astragalus

Astragalus is a popular herb used in Chinese medicine, usually alongside other herbs to prevent colds and respiratory infections. Astragalus is also used for the following ailments:

congestive heart failure   kidney disease

chronic fatigue syndrome   allergies

cancer   control of blood sugar levels

Rhodiola

Rhodiola is a plant mainly found in Europe and Asia. It is known to stabilize body functions and prevent stress-induced hormonal changes. Rhodiola is also used for the following ailments:

anxiety   fatigue   depression

stress   diabetes   cancer

Enhanced Amino Formula

What makes Synergy unique is that they have created their very own Amino acid formula, which contains high levels of antioxidant. Not only does it detoxify the body, but it also contains anti-aging properties. The Amino Acid formula gives the immune system a big boost and assists the T cells with the elimination of the herpes virus hiding in the spine.

Tribulus

Tribulus is an herb that has been used in China and India for hundreds of years and is known to improve athletic performance. Tribulus has been used as an aphrodisiac and is used to treat many sexual problems. It is also used for the following ailments:

cancer   pain   inflammation

blood pressure   kidney stones

Lysine

Lysine is an essential amino acid which supports the immune system. It's important for calcium absorption and cardiovascular function. It is often used to help prevent herpes outbreaks.

Lysine is also used for the following ailments:

cancer   anxiety   acne

digestion   diabetes

Below is a link to buy products from Synergy.

https://www.synergy-pharmaceuticals.com/

Testimonials

Below are just a few of the testimonials attesting to the effectiveness of their products. Their website has many more testimonials.

"Hope you are well and OK as well as the staff at Synergy Pharmaceutical. Just to let you know I had my blood test done.

The results…. Negative. Thank you so much all of you. It's peace of mind to know I'm free from this virus. I have recommended the product to three of my friends. All intrigued and want to try as I believe it's better I can be proof that you have cure. Thank you so much for continued rapport and feedback and guidance to my emails. Thank you so much, everyone." **NB**

"I have wonderful news!!! I took my blood test HSV IGG 1 and 2. The HSV1 IGG returned positive, but HSV 2 IGG returned negative (Hooray!!!). On the 27th of August will mark 90 days on the treatment. I am hopeful that HSV 1 will also become eradicated." **SK**

"I'd like to inform happy news. In last May, my IgM and IgG was negative and since last February I had no symptoms by now. And my doctor said he cannot believe this result and simultaneously he said it means virus does not exit in my body even if he cannot believe that. (In fact, all doctors in my country believe this hsv virus cannot be eliminated if once infected.) Anyway, thanks for this result." **KW**

"Unfortunately, my ex-husband left me with oral herpes, and I thought I would never have a love life again. I tried two other treatments with no success. When I found these pills, I took a leap of faith and did the treatment for 7 months. I just took my test, and it all came back negative!!!!! I'm fighting back tears as I type this testimonial. You can be free and healed from herpes. This is not a scam; it's real!" After using Synergy for 7 months, I have tested negative for hsv1. I am beyond enthused and so appreciative of the whole Synergy team. I feel like I have my life back. I no longer feel hopeless & alone. I want to thank the Synergy team for their exceptional customer service skills and thorough explanations whenever addressing my concerns. I also appreciate them keeping my privacy. I encourage anyone feeling hesitant or skeptical about trying Synergy or sticking

with the protocol to do it. It is so worth it in the end. The team
helps you along your healing journey. I was suicidal and hated
myself for contracting such a nightmare. I felt absolutely
disgusting. It was such a burden for me. I felt absolutely
helpless with the frequent symptoms. Trust the process & take
the advice of the Synergy team.” **AG**

“A huge thanks to you guys. It’s been such a turnaround for me.
I got the negative results back I was waiting for finally. It took a
little longer than I had hoped but you know I got there. One
thing I would suggest to other people is to watch the foods
cause they’re a major issue. For me it was the beer and nuts;
they were triggering things off but once I cut them out things
moved faster.” EV

“Product works wonders. I was diagnosed with HSV1 in my
genital area due to a previous relationship. I’ve used this for 6
months, had some pretty decent outbreak at the second month.
Lasted for over a week. Had the checkup probably two months
ago that came back negative to both HSV1 and HSV2. Very
happy with this product.” **DR**

Pros & Cons

There are many pros to buying this product. Firstly, the price is
reasonable, so you don’t really have anything to lose. If you are
not one of the few that are cured, then you still have access to
vitamins that will boost your immune system. Secondly, the
price is low in comparison to other herbs and other alternative
treatments for herpes. Customer service is great. They reply to
you in a timely manner via email, with lengthy replies, showing
their concern for your health.

The only con is that their success rate is not 100%. To increase
your chances of being among the 70% who have achieved
success, first implement the last method that we describe in this
book.

A New Product in America: Herpesyl

What is it?

Herpesyl contains 26 natural ingredients, all combined in one bottle. It eliminates the herpes virus using a two-step process. First, it gets rid of the virus from the brain. The brain, in turn, sends a signal to the body to boost the immune system.

The bottle contains 60 capsules and lasts one month, as the company recommends that you take two a day. It's relatively cheap in comparison to Dr. Sebi's products. It sells for $69 a bottle (at the time of this writing). Discounts are offered if you buy more than one bottle, and it comes with a 60-day money back guarantee.

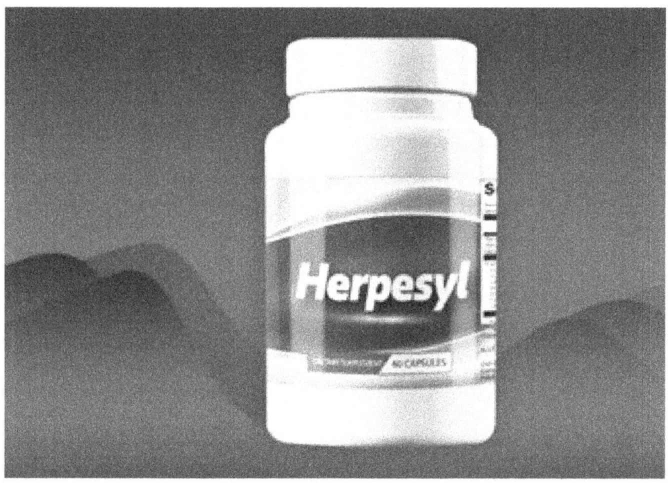

Ingredients

Below are some of the main ingredients used to make Herpesyl.

- **Graviola Extract:** Graviola is a plant found in the Americas and in the Caribbean. Because it contains a lot of antioxidants, it is known to offer a powerful boost to the immune system. Its antiviral properties aid in eliminating the virus from the body.

- **Tumeric:** Turmeric is a popular spice that some use to color their rice yellow and is known for its ability to fight inflammation. In Herpesyl, it plays a major role in eliminating the herpes virus.

- **Shitake Mushroom:** Though often used in cooking, Shitake is a popular mushroom used in Chinese medicine to fight fungal and viral infections. Shitake has been found to reverse the damage (in the brain) caused by the herpes virus.

- **Burdock Root:** Burdock root acts as a blood purifier, cleansing the blood of the herpes virus. Like Graviola, it is an antioxidant that strengthens the immune system and has anti-inflammatory properties as well.

- **Quercetin seeds:** Quercetin is another antioxidant that, when used in the Herpesyl formula, inhibits the HSV protein. It is also known for its anti-cancer properties.

- **Vitamin C:** Vitamin C helps to boost the immune system and aids the body in the event of an outbreak. Working alongside Vitamin E and Selenium, the Vitamin C pushes the virus out of the brain cells.

Where do I buy it?

Unfortunately, there are many dummy websites out there attempting to impersonate the company. Herpesyl does have a website (https://herpesyl.com/report), but it was down for a while. Other websites with the name herpesyl are not authentic. Also, stores like Walmart, Amazon, and Ebay also have products that are purportedly Herpesyl. However, upon close examination, you will see that the ingredients are different. You will also notice that above the word 'Herpesyl', you will see the name of a company other than Herpesyl.

So, how do you know if you have the right product? You MAY be able to find the authentic formula on Ebay but need to make sure that the following address is listed on the bottle.

37 Invernes Dr. E #100, Englewood, CO 80112

To ensure that you purchase the correct bottle, you can visit *buygoods.com* or call them at 1-302-200-3480. Their office hours are Monday through Friday, from 10 a.m. to 7 p.m. EST. Buygoods works as a third party selling the original product for Herpesyl Inc.

Pros & Cons

As with Synergy, the pros outweigh the cons. You have little to risk by buying this product. It's relatively inexpensive and offers a money back guarantee. If you are not one of the few that are cured, then you still have access to the various herbs that will boost your immune system. As for the cons, in my opinion, there are none.

Glad Tidings from the Mideast: The Hekmac Center

What does Hekmac Center have to offer?

Hekmac Center is a company based in Dubai, United Arab Emirates, which offers a variety of herbal products for different ailments, such as multiple sclerosis, respiratory disorders, Parkinson's disease, and herpes. In addition to packages for the aforementioned illnesses, they also sell natural supplements for other conditions like insomnia, migraine, and anxiety.

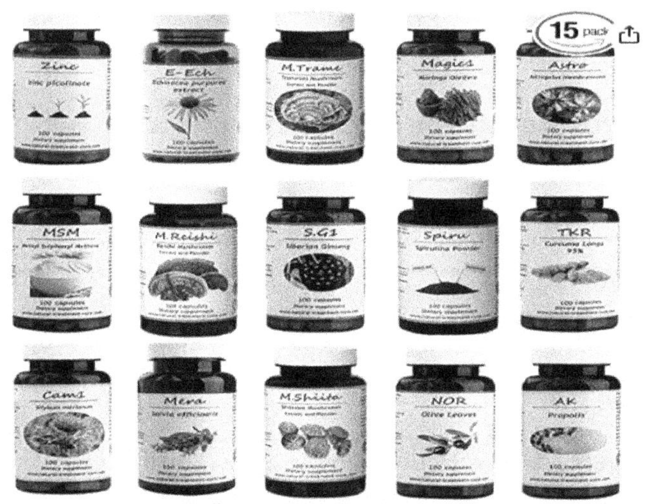

Ingredients

The package they offer for eradicating the herpes virus from the system consists of 15 different herbal products, all designed to be used synchronously. The package sells for $1500 (at the time of this writing). Some of the main herbs used are:

- **Curcumin:** Curcumin is the main active compound found in turmeric, a popular spice that some use to color their rice yellow. It's known for its anti-inflammatory properties and aids in reducing the effects of cancer, Alzheimer's, and heart disease.

- **Shitake:** Shitake is a popular mushroom recognized for its antiviral and antibacterial properties.   Its role in this formula is to prevent the herpes virus from entering the cells.

- **MSM (Methyl Sulfonyl Methane):** MSM is an anti-inflammatory often used to treat arthritis. Additionally, it is used for gastrointestinal disorders and to fight viruses.

- **Propolis:** Propolis is the bee glue that holds beehives together. Propolis contains flavonoids that function as antioxidants which lower your chances of getting cancer and heart disease. With herpes, it is said to reduce the viral load and prevent future outbreaks.

- **Moringa Oleifera:** Moringa is a plant found in India and has been used for thousands of years to treat ailments. It is known to activate cellular immunity in herpes sufferers. Other benefits of Moringa are that it reduces inflammation, lowers cholesterol levels, and lowers blood sugar levels.

- **Echinacea:** Often used with Vitamin C, Echinacea has been known to give a big immunity boost. It is a popular plant that Native Americans used to treat many different illnesses. Other benefits derived from

Echinacea are that it protects against cancer, treats
skin diseases, and lowers blood sugar levels.

- **Reishi Mushroom:** Like Shitake, Reishi is a popular
  mushroom known to fight viruses, bacteria, and
  cancer cells as well. It is known to slow down the
  replication of the herpes virus. Other benefits of
  Reishi are that it reduces risk of heart disease and
  diabetes.

- **Zinc:** If the body is deficient of Zinc, then herpes
  sufferers will have more outbreaks. In addition to
  boosting the immune system and thus preventing
  outbreaks, Zinc is known to accelerate wound healing,
  treat acne, and decrease inflammation.

Hekmac's herpes treatment package can be purchased at the
link below.

https://www.hekmac.com/en/shop2/herpes-simplex-virus-
hsv1-hsv2-supplements-copy/

Testimonials

Testimonials posted on their website include screenshots of
Whatsapp messages between Hekma Center and the customer
as well as before and after test results. Below are some of the
testimonials that can be found on Trustpilot.

"I can't say enough good things about Hekma Center. Dr Miriam is wonderful and answered all my questions via email. The products are excellent quality. I am age fifty and I now look and feel twenty years younger. My blood work is perfect. If you want perfect health please do not hesitate to contact Hekma Center. My only regret is that it took me so long to find them. Wonderful 5 star company. I can't say enough good things about Hekma Center. Thank you. Changed my life."

"Dr Miriam helped me defeat the HSV1 virus in 50 days. The diet was not easy but you get used to it after 1 week. It'll all be worth at the end of process! so, just be patient and keep communicating with Dr miriam if you have any concerns. I will definitely come back and recommend to my people I care about."

"I have suffered of HSV for 5 years, never thought that i will live without it until finding Hekma center. They have changed my life, finally, i am HSV free after 100 days of their fantastic plan."

"Hello, I am beyond thankful and grateful with this company Hekma Center, I had been contagious with this virus for about 20 years yes 20 years I thought that I would never get cured specially since this virus really was acting up in my body. It was really bad so many outbreaks and nonstop symptoms. I am 43 years old and I got divorced last year 2021 And I really thought I wasn't going to be able to date again since I felt dirty and fake. I am very surprised with the professionalism of the staff never but ever were unprofessional and I asked so many questions sometimes it was ridiculous but they were walking right beside me. On April 18, 2022 I started the process with the supplements and all the steps. After I was almost done with the 50 days I took a wrong test IgG test instead of the PCR and it came back positive. I told the staff and they told me I was supposed to do the PCR test and explained me the reason behind it. I went and I took the PCR test and it came back negative !!!!!!! Thank you God for giving me my health back. Thank you Hekma for exist, you gave me a second chance."

Pros and Cons

Hekmac boasts a 95% success rate in eliminating the herpes virus from the system. As for the five percent that have not been successful, they allege that it is because they have not followed instructions properly. As for the cons, it is extremely expensive.

An Approach Rarely Thought Of: Seeking Forgiveness

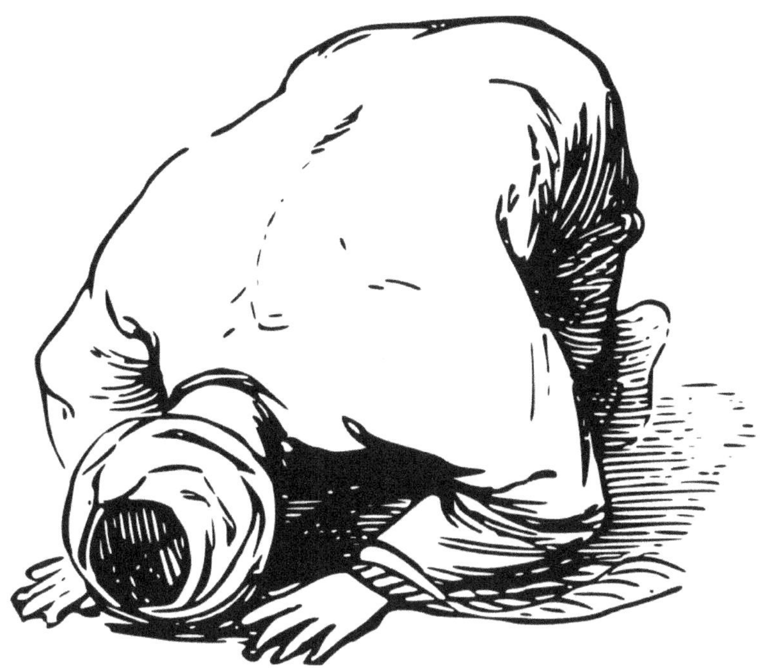

Seek Forgiveness

Seek forgiveness? What do you mean by seek forgiveness? Who do I have to apologize to? And for what? I haven't done anything wrong! These may be some questions going through your mind as you read these words.

By 'seek forgiveness', we mean to ask the One who made our bodies to forgive us for any possible misuse of it that may have resulted in contracting the herpes virus.

While we can't assume that *every* case of herpes is due to fornication or adultery, sometimes that is indeed the case. A person may have contracted it from sleeping around, while married or unmarried. Promiscuity has become rampant today, to the extent that people now look at someone who refrains from such deviant acts as the odd ball. Negative peer pressure prevails. People feel that if society says fornication is okay **today**, then it is. But who should we obey- the Creator or creation? What do the Holy Books have to say about fornication and adultery?

In the Bible, it says:

"Flee from sexual immorality. Every other sin a person commits is outside the body, but the sexually immoral person sins against his own body. Or do you not know that your body is a temple of the Holy Spirit within you, whom you have from God? You are not your own, for you were bought with a price. So, glorify God." (Corinthians 6:18-20)

"Know ye not that the unrighteous shall not inherit the kingdom of God? Be not deceived: neither fornicators, nor idolaters, nor adulterers, nor effeminate, nor abusers of themselves with mankind." (Corinthians 6:9-11)

And in the Quran, it says:

"And do not approach unlawful sexual intercourse. Indeed, it is ever an immorality and is evil as a way." (Quran 17:32)

In conjunction with the above verses, the last prophet, Muhammad (Peace and blessings be upon him, upon Prophet

Jesus, and on all the other prophets) had the following to say about unlawful intercourse:

He (peace be upon him) also said: "**Whenever adultery becomes a widespread phenomenon among certain people, death will spread among them.**" (Reported by Malik.)

In reflecting on the latter statement, a prediction made over 1400 years, we see that sexually transmitted diseases like AIDS, is a major cause of death today. An accurate, divinely inspired prediction! In 2020, nearly 1 million people died worldwide because of AIDS.

Your Body Has a Purpose

In today's changing society, the motto is, 'It's my body, I can do with it as I want.' But can you really…………without facing consequence? Consequences in this world and consequences in the Hereafter. Your body doesn't belong to you. Our bodies are a loan from the Creator, the Most High. The One who created the sun, the moon, the stars, the heavens, and the earth and all contained therein. We should do with it as **HE** pleases and not as we please!

Yes, we do have free will, but what we decide will either be **for** us *or* **against** us.

The earth doesn't belong to us. We have only been allowed to walk on it for a specified time. Our bodies were made with dirt (clay) and will return to dirt (in the grave) sooner than we think. The only thing that will remain when we die will be our deeds. That car that you owned will be sold or given to someone else.

Your clothes will be given away. Even your name won't follow you. You will be referred to during the burial as 'the body'. We will be held accountable for **every single thing** that we have done with our bodies. What we have allowed our ears to hear……what we have allowed our eyes to see……what we have allowed our hands to do…...what we have allowed our private parts to commit.

The earth belongs to the One who created it- God, the Most High. How would you feel if someone came into the house that belongs to you and did whatever they wanted to do, against your wishes? They went into your refrigerator and took out whatever they wanted. They slept in your bed without your permission. Would you allow it? Would you be happy with them? We should respect and walk on the earth that has been loaned to us in a dignified, obedient manner. In the way that is pleasing to God, the One who designed it.

Our bodies have a purpose. A house has a purpose. Its purpose is to provide shelter for us. A pen has a purpose. It's to write with. A phone has a purpose. Its purpose is to communicate with. How can a complex being- a human being- NOT have a purpose? What would you say if someone told you that Bill Gates didn't know why he designed Microsoft? Or Steve Jobs why he designed the iPhone or that the iPhone had no purpose? Does *not* the Creator know *why* he created man?

Everything that has been created, whether human or inanimate object, has a purpose and should be used according to rules set out by the creator of that object. If used in any other way, it won't last. If you used the mouse of a computer to scrub the wall, you would destroy it- both the mouse and the wall. The same can be said with the human body. If used in a way other than that designed and desired by the Creator, it will be destroyed.

'So, why am I here?' one might ask. As stated in the following verse of the Holy Quran, God created us so that we can worship Him and Him alone.

"And I (Allah) created not the jinn and mankind except that they should worship Me (Alone)." (Quran 51:56)

The concept of worship in Islam is a comprehensive one. It entails doing all the things that God loves- among the obligatory things as well as voluntary things and refraining from doing things displeasing to Him, such as murder, stealing, fornication and adultery. Once someone understands that the reason for their existence is to worship the One who created them, they will totally submit to the rules laid out by the Creator. Sexual promiscuity and the diseases resulting therefrom will then be a non-issue.

Life is indeed a test to see if we will fulfill the purpose for which we have been created or not. It has its ups and downs, but we must keep to the goal until we reach the finish line.

How Can Seeking Forgiveness Help Me

So, how can seeking forgiveness help me? And how do I go about doing it?

The Prophet Muhammad (Peace and blessings of God be upon him) said that **"every disease has a cure; if a cure is applied to the disease, it is relieved by the permission of Allah Almighty**." This statement was made more than 1400 years ago, knowing that in the future fornication would become rampant and thus, disease as well. The One who allowed the disease to happen to you – the Creator- can guide you to a cure. If we seek His forgiveness, He will help us. There have been stories of people making umrah (the minor pilgrimage to Makka, Saudi Arabia) and being cured from diseases like cancer and then returning with doctors unable to find a trace of the illness. *

The first step to asking God for forgiveness is to prostrate before your Lord (as in the picture on the preceding pages) and ask Him to forgive you and guide you. Then acknowledge the fact that there is no deity worth of worship except God (known as Allah), the One and Only, who has no sons nor daughters and that His last messenger is Prophet Muhammad (Peace and blessings of God be upon him). Once a person utters this testimony of faith, they have entered into the folds of Islam and ALL their sins will be wiped away.

"Prophet Muhammad (Peace and blessings of God be upon him) said: **'If a person accepts Islam, such that his Islam is good, Allah will decree reward for every good deed that he did before, and every bad deed that he did before will be erased.''**

To learn more about Islam, you can visit the following site. www.islam-guide.com

Pros & Cons

What do you have to lose by trying this approach? Nothing. What do you have to gain? Everything!

---

*See 'Allah Removes the Cancer-True Story' on YouTube

*Also, visit the following link to read about a Bosnian man cured after making hajj (major pilgrimage).

https://ilmfeed.com/bosnian-man-cured-tumor-went-hajj-drank-zamzam-water/

Methods to Control the Herpes Virus

If, somehow, you are still not convinced that there **really is** a cure for herpes and you just want to prevent frequent outbreaks, there are many things that you can do or take.

- **Raw Food Diet:** Some people swear that a raw food diet works to treat many ailments, from diabetes to cancer. A raw food diet consists of eating only fresh vegetables and fruits and abstaining from eating anything cooked. In addition to vegetables and fruits, smoothies are also made. This diet may last from several weeks to a couple of months.

- **Oregano Oil:** Many are probably familiar with the smell of oregano, the spice that is used in making pizza. Oregano Oil is extracted from a flowering plant native to Europe. Aside from its use in the kitchen to flavor food, it has many benefits. It is a natural antibiotic and powerful antioxidant and can be used to treat yeast infections as well as speed up the healing process of herpes sores.

- **Lysine**: Lysine is a must-have for anyone suffering from herpes. Taken regularly, Lysine can help prevent outbreaks by blocking the production of Arginine. Herpes sufferers should be careful to avoid eating too many foods rich in Arginine as they may trigger an outbreak. Lysine is also known to block stress response receptors, thus decreasing anxiety.

- **Reishi Mushroom**: Like Shitake, Reishi is a popular mushroom known to fight viruses, bacteria, and cancer cells as well. It is known to slow down the replication of the herpes virus. Other benefits of Reishi are that it reduces risk of heart disease and diabetes.

- **Ozone Therapy**: Ozone therapy is popular in some European countries, such as Turkey, Spain, England, and Greece. The use of ozone dates back to 1856 when it was used to disinfect instruments. It was also used to kill bacteria and viruses found in water. Ozone therapy entails hooking a person up to an IV, then extracting their blood in a sterile vacuum ozone bottle and then giving it back to the person after it has been ozonized. In Turkey, Ozone Therapy treatment is relatively cheap (usually under $50), depending on the dosage. Natural Life Clinic (Doğal Hayat Polikliniği) in Ankara, Turkey treats herpes sufferers using Ozone Therapy. Their website is listed below.

  https://www.dogalhayat.com.tr/

- **Ayuverda Medicine:** Ayuverda is an alternative medicine practice which has been in existence in India for thousands of years. It is based on the presumption that disease is caused by an imbalance in a person's consciousness. Not only does Ayuverda treat different ailments using herbal medicines but also by suggesting special diets and incorporating yoga and meditation in the client's daily routine. Among the many diseases treated using Ayuverdic medicine is herpes. Biogetica, a company based in India, offers a product they say has shown to completely suppress the herpes virus. They have clinical trials to support their claims and offer a 90 money back guarantee on their products. Their website is https://www.biogetica.com/is-herpes-treatment-a-herpes-cure

- **Neem**:   Long used in Indian medicine, neem oil has many benefits. It is excellent for the skin and is known to have anti-aging properties. Aside from using neem oil to treat acne, neem oil is also used to speed up the healing of herpes cold sores. As for the leaves of the neem plant, they can be used as a preventative measure to ward off potential outbreaks.

- **Olive Leaf:**   Known for its popularity in the Mideastern diet, the olive has many benefits in its various forms- as a leaf, oil, and extract. Its main ingredient, oleuropein, contains powerful antioxidant and anti-inflammatory properties. It has been used successfully in fighting cancer, heart disease, diabetes, and even herpes.

Conclusion

The purpose of this book was to introduce you to remedies that you may have never heard of. It is not intended to be used to diagnose and treat ailments. It is upon you to conduct thorough research of the methods shared here, some of which I myself have personally tried.

There is a cure for everything, whether we have discovered it or not. The ultimate decision is up to the Creator to guide us to that cure and then decree it for us.

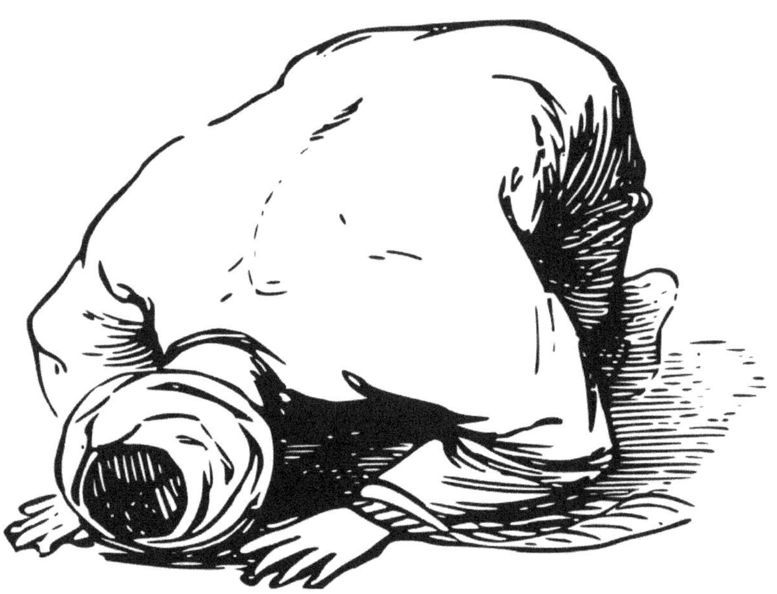

About the Author

After suffering from symptoms of cancer, I tried various natural methods to cure it. I went to a Chinese doctor in the States as well as one in UK for acupuncture. I found that instead of reducing the pain, the acupuncture actually caused more pain, so I stopped that treatment. I also traveled to Turkey and while there, had leech therapy, which I found left me with a refreshed feeling and may have contributed to stopping the spread of the cancer. Though I had cancer for three years, once I was finally diagnosed (third year), I was still at Stage One. Thank God. I also had Vitamin C therapy and Oxygen therapy in Turkey. Another alternative treatment I tried was ruqya and cupping, which always had a direct impact on my symptoms, causing them to decrease. Despite trying various natural methods, I finally succumbed to getting an operation to have the tumor removed but did not get radiation nor chemotherapy (though radiation was recommended). To maintain a healthy lifestyle and to keep the cancer from returning (now 2 years later), I pray, firstly, and then exercise and take Graviola, Vitamin C, and garlic daily.

I also had herpes for 12 years, which I contracted from my ex-husband. To completely eradicate the virus from my system, I firstly improved my relationship with my Creator (page 39). Secondly, after using Herpesyl (page 31) for 6 months, alongside Synerygy (page 26) products, I finally received negative test results from the hospital and am symptom free. I can eat all the trigger foods that I once could not eat, but nothing happens. Thank God.

*Please note, it appears that Synergy is out of business. Sadly, they were a great support. All hope is not lost though. I had used their product for years actually, but I did not receive negative results until I tried Herpesyl alongside it.

Glossary of Arabic Terms

Allah   This is an Arabic term and refers to the One and Only God, the Creator of the heavens and earth. Contrary to what some may mistakenly believe, it does not mean a separate god. Allah has no partners nor offspring and is not in need of His creation. Nor does He resemble His creation in any way. He is the Almighty, the Wise, and to Him we return.

Jinn   Invisible creatures made of fire. Some are good, and some are bad (demons). Some may call them ghosts, but they are not the souls of the dead. There is a chapter in the Quran that talks about them.

Mosque   A place of worship where Muslims pray.

Muhammad   The last prophet, born in Makka 570 A.D. He spread the teachings of Islam, the fastest growing religion in the world.

Quran   The last divine revelation. It is read by Muslims all over the world.

Shahada   This is the testimony of faith. It consists of one statement, said in Arabic, and with this statement, a person becomes a Muslim.

HOW DO I BECOME MUSLIM?

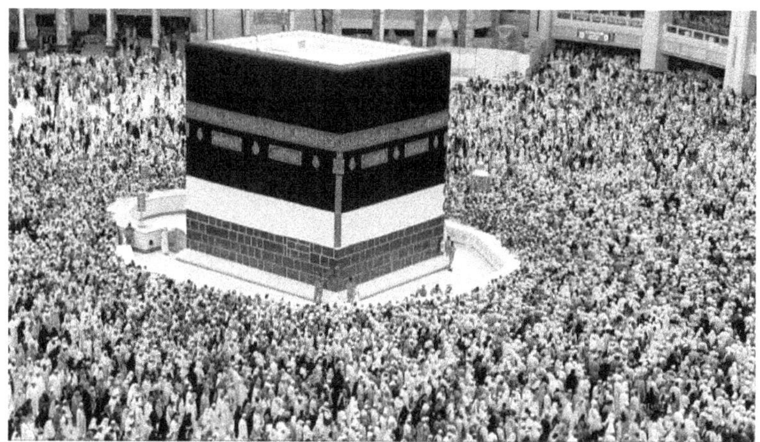

You simply say the testimony of faith.

The Shahadah (testimony of faith): Ash hadu an laa ilaha illa Allah wa ash hadu anna Muhammadan rasoolullah (Arabic)

I bear witness that there is no god worthy of worship except Allah, and I bear witness that Muhammad is the messenger of Allah. (English translation)

Lysine-Rich Foods

- Meat- red meat & poultry
- Cheese, especially parmesan & Low-fat Ricotta cheese
- Certain fish, such as cod, tuna, & sardines
- Milk
- Eggs.
- Soybeans, particularly tofu, isolated soy protein, and defatted soybean flour.
- Canned navy beans
- Spirulina
- Fenugreek seed
- King crab

Food	Arginine	Lysine
Soy protein isolate	6670	5327
Peanuts, dry-roasted	2832	850
Almonds, dry-roasted	2444	563
Black beans, boiled	549	608
Milk, 2% (cow)	94	276
Egg, hard-boiled	755	904
Beef, chuck, braised	2054	2748

Adopted from the US Department of Agriculture National Nutrient Database

Bibliography

https://www.healthline.com/nutrition/astragalus#dosage

https://www.healthline.com/nutrition/rhodiola-rosea#TOC_TITLE_HDR_8

https://www.synergy-pharmaceuticals.com/testimonials/

https://www.synergy-pharmaceuticals.com/

https://www.verywellfit.com/tribulus-benefits-uses-tips-and-more-89589

https://www.healthline.com/nutrition/tribulus-terrestris#TOC_TITLE_HDR_8

7 Amazing Benefits of Lysine | Organic Facts

https://www.globenewswire.com/fr/news-release/2021/04/23/2216179/0/en/Herpesyl-Customer-Reviews-2021-Ingredients-Benefits-Side-Effects-User-Reviews-Reviewed-By-ConsumersCompanion.html

https://www.outlookindia.com/outlook-spotlight/herpesyl-reviews-is-it-legit-or-scam-shocking-ingredients--news-205177

https://ipsnews.net/business/2020/10/19/herpesyl-reviews-user-exposed-truth-must-read-before-buy/

https://dailyiowan.com/2022/01/21/herpesyl-reviews-shocking-read-this-ingredients-report-now-before-buying/

https://www.hekmac.com/en/shop2/herpes-simplex-virus-hsv1-hsv2-supplements-copy/

https://www.trustpilot.com/review/hekmacenter.com

https://rosewellness.com/mushrooms-boost-immunity/

https://www.webmd.com/diet/health-benefits-reishi-mushrooms#1

Propolis: Health Benefits, Uses, Dosage, and More (webmd.com)

https://www.webmd.com/diet/health-benefits-msm#1

https://www.healthline.com/nutrition/9-oregano-oil-benefits-and-uses#1.-Natural-antibiotic

https://www.dogalhayat.com.tr/tr/tedaviler/geleneksel-tedaviler/ozon-tedavisi/ozon-tedavisi-nasil-yapilir

https://www.hopkinsmedicine.org/health/wellness-and-prevention/ayurveda

https://www.thehealthsite.com/ayurveda/us-grants-patent-to-ayurvedic-remedy-for-herpes-765419/

https://www.webmd.com/diet/health-benefits-olive-leaf-extract#1

https://www.openbible.info/topics/fornication

https://www.kingjamesbibleonline.org/Bible-Verses-About-Fornication/

https://www.unaids.org/en/resources/fact-sheet

https://sunnah.com/nasai:4998

https://ilmfeed.com/bosnian-man-cured-tumor-went-hajj-drank-zamzam-water/

https://drsebiscellfood.com/pages/drsebi

https://www.vibe.com/features/viva/dr-sebi-reportedly-dies-in-custody-443391/

https://en.wikipedia.org/wiki/Alfredo_Bowman

https://www.youtube.com/watch?v=y4J8BxbqXOA

https://www.youtube.com/watch?v=sq2OUdle6Bg

https://miskawaanhealth.com/cancer/ozone-therapy/

https://academic.oup.com/painmedicine/article/11/3/443/1886470

https://www.healthline.com/health/what-is-leech-therapy#medical-applications

https://www.leechestherapy.com/about-leeches/benefits

https://www.healthline.com/health/what-is-leech-therapy#medical-applications

https://healthandvitalitycenter.com/treatments/vitamin-c-iv/

https://www.sciencedirect.com/science/article/pii/S0753332222002967

https://www.hopkinsmedicine.org/health/wellness-and-prevention/acupuncture

https://www.medicalnewstoday.com/articles/156488

https://www.mayoclinic.org/tests-procedures/acupuncture/about/pac-20392763

https://www.ncbi.nlm.nih.gov/pmc/articles/PMC2642987/

https://www.ncbi.nlm.nih.gov/pmc/articles/PMC9676348/#:~:text=Surveys%20showed%20that%20cupping%20for,after%20the%20moving%20cupping%20therapy.

https://www.masnad.com.au/hijama-and-diabetes/

https://www.ncbi.nlm.nih.gov/pmc/articles/PMC5103544/

https://www.ncbi.nlm.nih.gov/pmc/articles/PMC3151529/#:~:text=Wet%20cupping%20is%20a%20traditional,zoster%20compared%20with%20western%20medication.

https://www.webmd.com/balance/cupping-therapy

https://www.webmd.com/cancer/graviola-cancer-overview

https://www.youtube.com/watch?v=V2TkcN49q5o&t=70s

https://www.medicalnewstoday.com/articles/319720#potential-health-benefits

https://www.healthline.com/health/boswellia#cancer

https://www.medicalnewstoday.com/articles/326599#how-to-take

https://www.healthline.com/nutrition/top-10-evidence-based-health-benefits-of-turmeric

https://www.hopkinsmedicine.org/health/wellness-and-prevention/turmeric-benefits